Your
Little Book
of
Spiritual
Knowledge

Your Spirit, Your Life Series

Book 2

Mark W. Neville

Dedication

To you and all the living.

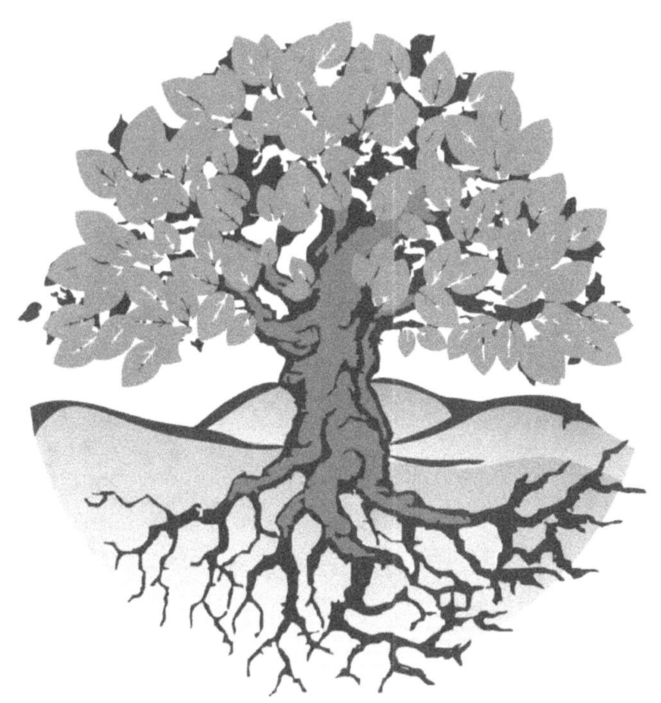

Contents

Acknowledgements

Deep gratitude flows from my heart to Lisa—
my best friend, lover, and wife. Without her this book
would not be. I would not be.
Heart-felt thanks also goes to my many hospice patients
and private clients. This book would not be without them.
They have been and remain my best teachers.
I have also been blessed with an abundance of professors,
mentors, and colleagues—too many to list here. For them
also my heart swells with gratitude.
Thank you!

PREFACE

An Invitation

Wonder of wonders! Mystery of mysteries! You are alive rather than not!

Let the profound mystery of this mere fact sink in: You. Are. Alive!

You aren't just rare. Like a meteor, you happen once. You are a once-in-forever, here-and-gone human being of inestimable worth.

And you are not alone. You. Are. Alive. With Others!

Never again take your life or anyone else's for granted—human or otherwise. Never again take your relationships for granted.

A Question

Now wonder about this: *What* makes you and others alive? God? A chemical process? Something else?

This little book explores a different answer to that question. What makes you and others alive is a *phenomenon of nature*, a *natural force*. The natural force that lights a lightbulb is electricity. The natural force in magnetite stones that attract iron is magnetism. And the natural force that makes you and every living thing alive is spirit.

As you see the effects of and feel the natural forces of electricity and magnetism, so you see the natural energy of spirit with your own eyes and feel it inside you. You experience spirit first-hand. You see the difference between a tree that is spirited and alive and another that's not. You feel that you are spirited and alive rather than not. Sometimes you feel more spirited than other times.

In this little book, spirit is not a religious concept or belief. Instead of *capital 'S' Spirit*, it is about lower *case 's' spirit*. This book does not refer to spirit as a divine being like the Holy Spirit, Great Spirit, Universe, or a Higher Power. Neither does it refer to your soul, a spark of God, Higher Self, or anything eternal in you that survives death.

Rather than asserting anything about the ultimate

origin or nature of your spirit—whether it's God, a chemical process, or something else—this little book points out the *natural phenomenon* and *force* of spirit in *this* physical realm of your experience. It directs your attention to it, shows it to you, and describes it in detail.

 It starts by describing a problem, a *spiritual* problem.

INTRODUCTION

A Spiritual Problem

Here's the thing: you know about your *body*.
You've learned basic biology. You learned the
names of your body parts when you were a child.
You know what they do. You know about germs,
handwashing, cuts, twisted ankles, broken bones,
and first aid. You know about diseases, physicians,
hospitals, antibiotics, and pain meds.

You know about your *mind*. You've learned basic
psychology. You've heard of Freud, ego, id,
superego, and complexes. You've heard of Jung,
Adler, and Frankl and other psychologists.

You know about different functions of your mind:
memory, imagination, language processing,
problem-solving, dreaming, and more. You know
about anxiety, depression, and other mental
illnesses; antidepressants, anti-anxiety medications,
psychotherapists, and psychiatrists.

But you probably don't know about your *spirit*. You have no basic spiritual knowledge. You can't name the parts or functions of your spirit. You don't know when your spirit is healthy or not.

You don't know how to take care of your spirit or heal it when it's sick, wounded, or broken. You don't know of therapies for your spirit or professionals to see for diseases of your spirit.

You have a *spiritual* problem, and it's not your fault. Your parents didn't teach you about spirit, neither did your schoolteachers. They couldn't.

There is no publicly shared body of knowledge to teach. There are no sciences devoted to studying the natural phenomenon of spirit. There are no therapies for healing your spirit.

Why? Why didn't your parents and schoolteachers teach you about spirit? Why are there no sciences and therapies devoted to spirit?

It's a cultural thing with a history too long and complex to go into here. I tell that story in an upcoming book, *Re-Visioning Spiritual Knowledge: An Introduction to Thumology.* Suffice it to say here that the story is about belief in an invisible, divine, *capital 'S' Spirit* overshadowing knowledge of the *natural phenomenon* of spirit.

No, this book is not a critique of religion. It neither promotes nor disparages atheism or theism. It promotes attending to and learning about the natural phenomenon of spirit, your own and other's too.

Whether you're a believer, agnostic, or atheist, this little book is for you. Besides, knowing *why* you don't know *about* your spirit, doesn't teach you anything about spirit. It's time to change that. It's time for you to learn about your spirit and other's spirits too. Your life depends on it. So do the lives of others.

What You Gain from This Book

After reading this book you'll understand that if you know all there is to know about your body and mind, but know nothing about your spirit, you don't know what's most important to know about yourself. Nothing is more important than knowing your spirit.

Ignorance of spirit is far worse than any other kind of ignorance. Ignorance of spirit causes great harm to every living being on this planet. Until you know your spirit, you don't know yourself. Knowing your spirit is essential to knowing who you are and your reason for being alive.

After reading this book, you'll understand that if you take excellent care of your body and mind, but not your spirit, you're not caring for your most important part: your spirit. Nothing is more important than taking good care of your spirit. *Nothing.*

When your spirit is weak, sick, or wounded, so are your body and mind.

When your spirit is broken, you're at risk of dying.

Without spirit, your mind shuts down. Without spirit, your body is a cadaver.

Your spirit is your life. It's what makes you alive.

Where there is spirit, there is life. Where there is no spirit, there is no life.

Purpose of This Book

The purpose of this book is to introduce you to your own spirit. After reading and understanding this book, you will know what your spirit is and its basic anatomy. You will understand your desires, instincts, aspirations, emotions, moods, and inner knowing.

You will know that there is a reason for you being

alive. You will learn how to know and realize your reason for being alive—and nothing is more important for you to do than realize the purpose of your life.

You will—

- *learn basic spiritual exercises that will help you know and take good care of your spirit.*

- *learn how to know and fulfill your spirit's life-affirming desires and realize your dream.*

- *understand the spirits of others, not just of other humans, but of all living things.*

You'll have a basic understanding of different types of spirits. Understanding different spiritual types is essential to understanding your own personality and character as well as other's.

Your knowledge of spirit will increase your appreciation of your own life and the lives of others. You'll improve your life and live in a more life-affirming way. As you improve your own life, you will improve the lives of all others as well.

My Perspective

My perspective is holistic, spirit-focused, and Western-rooted.

I see you as a whole person: body, mind, and spirit. But you are more than body, mind, and spirit. You are holonic; that is, you are a whole, living human being with a distinct identity. Your identity as a whole is greater than the sum of your body, mind, and spirit, and all of your other smaller parts.

Just as every tree is a living whole, with a distinct identity that is greater than the sum of its roots, trunk, limbs, bark, leaves, and other smaller parts, so are you. Just as the smaller parts of a tree are themselves distinct wholes greater than the sum of their parts, so are your body, mind, and spirit. Every smaller part of you is a distinct whole that is greater than the sum of its parts.

Furthermore, a living tree is not an it-object isolated from everything around it. It's connected with the earth from which it grows. It's an outgrowth of the earth. A living tree is connected with and absorbs the water below in the earth and above that falls as rain. It's connected with the wind. It breathes. And it's connected with and absorbs the light of the sun. Just as a living tree is connected with and dependent on everything around it for its life, so are you.

In this book, you focus on one part of your whole self: your spirit. You learn about your spirit as a whole and its smaller parts. You also learn about how your spirit connects with others.

The view of spirit you learn here is rooted in Western culture, not Middle Eastern, Eastern, Native American, or African cultures. It's informed by the view of spirit found in the indigenous cultures of Greece, Rome, and the tribes of Northern Europe. Homer, Hesiod, the Greek lyric poets, dramatists, historians, and physicians, as well as Roman and Norse poets, inspire it. So do many modern philosophers, psychologists, writers, and poets.

Again, in this view, spirit is a natural phenomenon and force, like magnetism and electricity. It's the natural force that makes living things alive. Whatever is alive has spirit, including goddesses, gods, and other beings invisible to us. As long as something has spirit, it lives. When it expires, spirits out, it dies.

Overview

This little book has five parts.

Part One introduces you to your spirit. First, it describes what your spirit is not. Then it introduces you to a fundamental spiritual exercise. This essential exercise helps you know your own spirit firsthand. After introducing you to your spirit, this part describes in more detail the phenomenon of your spirit.

Part Two describes your spirit's anatomy. You know the basic anatomy of your body. It's time to know the basic anatomy of your spirit.

Part Three describes your spirit's health. You know about physical and mental health. It's time to learn about spiritual health and basic spiritual hygiene. In Part Three you learn five spiritual exercises for nurturing the health and well-being of your spirit.

Part Four you'll learn about spiritual disease and healing. In this part, you learn the seventh spiritual exercise presented in this book: Heart-Centered Self-Healing.

Part Five is about fulfilling the life-affirming desires of your heart. In this section, you learn how to know and realize your reason for being alive.

This book ends with a look forward at resources for learning more about your spirit and living a spirit-minded life. *The Thumotic Manifesto* is included as an appendix.

Thank You

Thank you for reading this far. I trust you'll enjoy and be enriched as you read the rest of this book.

As promised, Part One begins with describing what your spirit is not.

PART ONE: INTRODUCING YOUR SPIRIT

1- WHAT YOUR SPIRIT IS *NOT*

A Religious, Metaphysical Concept

Knowing your spirit begins with knowing what it is not. In this little book, your spirit is not viewed as a religious or metaphysical construct. You are certainly free to believe that your spirit is a religious or metaphysical thing. However, in this little book, your spirit is viewed differently.

It's not viewed as the Spirit of God, a spark of God, or God. You might well be filled with the Holy Spirit of God. You might be a spark of God trapped in a physical body. Or, you and everything else might actually be God. Those are different views from seeing your spirit as a natural phenomenon.

In this book, your spirit is also not your eternal soul or Higher Self. You might well have an eternal soul or Higher Self. It's not the concern of this book to confirm or deny that.

Here your spirit differs from your soul and Higher Self. Here your spirit is not "Spirit." It's not God's Holy Spirit in you. Neither is your spirit what makes you a "spiritual being having a human experience." Rather your spirit is what makes you a living human being.

This book isn't about you being an extraterrestrial soul who comes from a higher place, passes through this material world to learn lessons, and keeps reincarnating until to you return to your true home above.

In this book, you're fully human. You are more or less spirited, depending on your condition and circumstances. You're born, live, and die here. This is your home, at least for now.

A Psychological Construct

In this book, your spirit is not a psychological construct as conceived by Freud, Jung, Adler, or any other psychiatrist or psychologist. Your spirit is not your *psyche* or part of your *psyche*. It's different. While your soul or *psyche* continues to exist after you die and might reincarnate, your spirit doesn't. When you expire, that is, spirit-out, your spirit dissipates into the wind.

A Physical Construct

Magnetism and electricity are not just energy. Neither is your spirit. Just as magnetism and electricity are energy organized in specific ways, so is your spirit. Your spirit is energy organized in a particular way that makes you alive.

Your spirit is not reducible to a biological or chemical process. You're not alive because of the chemical process of your metabolism. Metabolism is a feature of being alive, not what makes you alive. Without spirit, you have no metabolism.

2- WHAT YOUR SPIRIT *IS*

A Natural Force

Your spirit is the natural force that makes you alive rather than not. It's the agent of your life.

Your life is a condition, time-period, narrative, and animating force. It's the condition of being alive. It's the time-period between your birthday and death day. It's a narrative, the story of your life, represented by the dash between your birth and death dates. It's all made possible because you have life in you. You have spirit.

Your spirit is centered between your breasts and behind your breastbone. It's the core, the heart of your being. You can become mentally aware of it with the following exercise.

Exercise #1: Your Basic Spiritual Exercise

Resources

You need nothing special to do this exercise. There is nothing to buy: no books, special clothing, jewelry, images, or paraphernalia. You already have everything you need.

You do not have to go to a special place. You can do this exercise anywhere. You do not have to do this exercise at a particular time. You can do it anytime.

You do not have to learn to sit a unique way or do anything out of the ordinary with your legs, hands, or posture. Any posture is fine.

Benefits

This exercise helps you learn to use your mind to serve your spirit. It heightens your mental awareness of your spirit. It affirms, heals, and strengthens your spirit. These benefits increase as you do this exercise on a regular basis.

Goal

The goal of this essential exercise is to be mindful of your own spirit with complete openness, full acceptance, and kind curiosity. Turning your mind's attention to your spirit and calmly holding it there with no expectations of outcomes is the only goal.

It's not the purpose of this exercise to feel calm and centered. The only goal is to simply be aware of your spirit, whatever its condition. However, one possible side-effect of this practice is feeling calmer and more centered.

What to Do

1. Close your eyes and cross your hands over your breastbone, the center of your chest.

2. Focus your mind's attention behind your breastbone. This is your heart, the core of your being. It's the center of your spirit. Smile at your own spirit. Actually smile.

3. Breathe in and smile into your heart; breathe out and smile out from your heart. As you breathe in mentally say to yourself, "I smile into my heart." As you breathe out say, "I smile out from my heart."

4. When your mind wanders, simply return your attention to your spirit in the heart of your chest. Breathe in and smile into your heart; breathe out and smile out from your heart.

5. Continue being mindful of your spirit for as long as you like. Stop when it feels right. It's that simple.

Beyond Your Spirit's Center

Although your spirit is centered in your heart, its circumference is currently unknown. Is your skin the boundary of your spirit? Or does your spirit extend beyond it? If it extends beyond your skin, how far? Is it infinite?

Did your spirit have a beginning? Did it exist before you were born? If it existed before you were born, where was it? Has it always existed? Is it eternal?

While many have beliefs, no one really knows the answers to these questions. We may never know because we're limited human beings and our knowledge is limited. It's okay to be at peace with unanswered questions.

What you do know is that your spirit is a smaller part of greater wholes. For example, the family you grew up in was a whole with its own distinct identity and spirit. So was the school you went to.

Your school had its own school spirit. Your spirit was part of it, and its spirit was part of you. It was unique, unlike any other school around.

If you participated in a sport, band, or club, then you know about *esprit de corps*. It's the spirit of a group that is a whole larger and other than you. With *esprit de corps* the group acts as a whole.

The community, town, or city you live in is a whole with its own distinct identity and spirit. Your spirit is part of that larger spiritual whole, and it is part of you. If you work for a company, it too is a whole with its own spirit. Your spirit is a smaller part of that company's spirit.

The state where you live has its own spirit of which yours is a smaller part. The same is true of the nation, hemisphere, planet, solar system, galaxy, and beyond. Your spirit is a small part of every greater spiritual whole beyond you.

You influence those greater spiritual wholes, and they influence you.

PART TWO: YOUR SPIRIT'S ANATOMY

3- YOUR INSTINCTS AND ASPIRATIONS

Your body has an anatomy, so does your spirit. Your spirit's anatomy includes its instincts, aspirations, emotions, moods, and inner-tutor.

Your Instincts

Your spirit makes you alive, and its instincts compel you to do what you need to do to stay alive.

To stay alive you must flee from, fight, or freeze in response to threats. You must also have shelter, work, eat, drink, rest, and sleep. Your spirit's instincts drive you to do these things and more to take good care of yourself, stay alive, and thrive.

Your Spirit's Life-Affirming Desires and Dream

Your spirit bears your reason for being alive. It carries the aspirations of your life: your dream and the life-affirming desires of your heart.

The original meaning of dream is not "sleeping vision." Etymologists don't know how dream came to refer to a sleeping vision. Dream is an Old English word that refers to *joy, mirth, noisy merriment, and music.*

Instead of a sleeping vision, a dream is a celebration. It's actual in-the-world joy and mirth expressed in noisy merriment and music. It's like a party.

Your Reason for Being Alive

Your reason for being alive is to realize your dream and joy. To know your joy, you must use your mind to attend to your spirit. Your spirit bears your dream, the joy you're here to realize. It takes time, quietness, attention, intention, and effort to become mentally aware of your dream.

When you engage in realizing your dream and joy, you feel in place, often lose track of time, and become one with what you're doing. You feel energized and glad afterward.

In Part Five of this little book, you receive specific guidance on how to become mentally aware of your dream. The point here is to know you have a dream. You need to become aware of it and how important it is to realize it.

Your dream tugs at your heart, and your heart's life-affirming desires stretch toward your dream. Your dream is your destiny to realize, and your life-affirming desires guide you in making it real.

Nothing, absolutely nothing is more critical for you to do than realize your dream and joy. It's the reason you're alive. It's what you're here to do.

You *must* realize your *joy. You need to. We all* need you to do what you're here to do. Realize the intention of your life. When you engage in realizing your joy, you fill us with joy too. Let *nothing* stop you from realizing your joy.

Know this: your spirit will nag you until you engage in realizing your dream. It will bother you until you do. You might even get physically sick or depressed if you resist your joy or get caught up in other distractions and neglect it.

Realizing your joy is your destiny. Your joy is calling you. Your spirit's relentless desire compels you to realize it. It's what you must do before you die. If you don't, you might die with genuine regrets.

4-YOUR EMOTIONS AND MOODS

Your Emotions

Your emotions are your spirit's acute responses to stimuli. They provide you with vital information about your circumstances and the health and wellbeing of your life.

Your spirit's emotions are stirred up, remain stirred up as long as the stimulus continues, and then resolve. They come and go and don't last long.

Two basic types of stimuli stir up your spirit's emotions: experienced-based and mind-based.

> *Experience-based* stimuli are in-the-world, external stimuli perceived through your five senses.

Mind-based stimuli are mental, internal stimuli like self-talk, memories, and imaginings.

Your spirit has ten basic emotional responses:

Fear is its response to threats, and *contentment* is its response to safety.

Anger is its response to being wronged, and *guilt* is its response to doing wrong.

Disappointment is your spirit's response to desire denied, and *gratitude* is its response to desire fulfilled.

Disgust is its response to what repels it, and *desire* is its response to what attracts it.

Sadness is your spirit's response to loss, and *gladness* is its response to gain.

Each one of your ten basic emotions vary in degrees of intensity. For example, your anger ranges from mild annoyance to complete outrage. Your gladness ranges from mild to ecstatic bliss. And so on for your eight other emotions.

Notice where you feel your emotions. Do you feel them in your head, between your ears? Probably not. You probably feel them in your heart, the center of your chest, and the surrounding area above and below it.

With some emotions, your spirit, also called your heart, contracts into hardness. With others, it softens. With some, it feels cold, with others hot. With still others, it expands either up into your throat and constricts it or into your face and drains or flushes it.

Sometimes it expands downward and fills your stomach with butterflies or ties it in knots. When it expands further down, your spirit engorges your genitalia with blood, heat, and wetness or contracts and shrivels them up. At times your emotions affect your bladder and bowels.

NOTE: Your spirit does not distinguish between experience-based and mind-based stimuli. For example, it responds with fear to both experience-based threats and mind-based self-talk, memories, and imaginings of threats.

Your Moods

Emotions are your spirit's acute responses. Moods are your spirit's chronic emotions. Whereas your emotions come and go over a short period, your moods last longer. It's as if the stimuli of moods prompt a prolonged rather than short response. The stimuli of moods are complex. Some are physical and related to changes in your body's chemistry.

What you eat and drink affects your mood.

Some stimuli are mental. Your attitudes, interpretations, opinions, and beliefs affect your mood. So do your self-talk, imaginings, and memories—especially when you ruminate. Other stimuli are social. For example, living with financial, food, housing, medical, and transportation insecurities affect your mood. So, does living with abuse and neglect.

Still, other stimuli are spiritual; that is, of your own or other's spirits. For example, practicing the essential mindfulness of spirit exercise described earlier affects your mood. So does interacting with someone who has a loving spirit or another who sucks the spirit and life out of you.

5- Your Inner-tutor, Greater Wholes, and types

Your Spirit's Knowing

You've experienced your heart telling you one thing and your head another. You know that inner conflict. It's the conflict between your spirit and mind.

Your spirit has its own cognizance. It's your heart knowledge, your inner knowing. It's wordless. Irrational. You just know without knowing how you know. You feel it. You feel it in your heart.

It's called intuition. "Intuition" comes from a Latin word that combines "inner" and "tutor." A tutor, in its original meaning, is a guardian of children. The tutor's primary responsibility is to keep the child safe. While keeping the child safe, the child also learns from the tutor by observing and asking questions.

Your spirit is your inner-tutor, your personal, inner guardian. It guards your life and helps keeps you safe.

As your inner-tutor, your spirit gives you that wordless sense that you're forgetting something, that you should take one route rather than another, that something has happened to someone you have a strong emotional connection with, and other matters that you know without knowing how you know them.

Perhaps you know from your own experience that you do well to heed your spirit's wordless inner knowing. In the conflict between your head and heart, you do well to go with your inner-tutor.

Your Spirit as a Smaller Part of Greater Wholes

The anatomy of your spirit is about the smaller parts of your spirit. But your spirit is also a whole with a distinct identity greater than the sum of its smaller parts.

As a whole, your spirit is also a smaller part of larger wholes: your family, community, school, business company, and more. In other words, your spirit is a smaller part of the anatomy of the larger spiritual wholes you participate in. Your own spirit influences the spirit of those larger wholes.

Your spirit influences the spirit of your family, community, school, company, state, country, and more. The healthier your spirit is, the healthier are the greater wholes it's a part of.

Likewise, the spirits of the larger wholes you participate in are aspects of your own spirit's anatomy. The spirits of the larger wholes you participate in are part of your own spirit's anatomy. They influence your own spirit. Their health influences yours.

A Taxonomy of Spiritual Types

Your spirit is of a particular type. It's similar to some and differs from others.

Whereas your emotions and moods are related in that they're both emotional responses, your spiritual type is not an emotional response. It's an inherent characteristic of your spirit.

Whereas your emotional responses are shorter and moods longer, the character of your spirit tends to be lifelong. Just as you experience your instincts, aspirations, emotions, moods, and inner knowing, you also experience different types of spirits.

When talking about the spiritual types of others, you might use heart, presence, or life as synonyms for the spirit of their character. For example, you know individuals who are consistently kind-hearted, great-spirited (their *presence* fills the room), or they suck the *life* right out of you and others they interact with.

Their spirit is of a particular type; your own spirit is of a particular kind too. Their spirit informs their personality; and yours informs your personality. There are many different types of spirits.

Listing the different types creates a taxonomy of spirits. I've coined many clinical terms for different spiritual types. They're listed in the *Thumotic Lexicon* in the back of my first book, *Re-Visioning Spirit: A Brief Introduction to Thumotics*. My upcoming book, *Re-Visioning Spiritual Knowledge An Introduction to Thumology*, will include an updated taxonomy of spirits.

Below is a short list of spiritual types in non-clinical language. Some might be familiar to you. Again, heart is a synonym for spirit.

Calm-spirited	High-spirited
Cold-hearted	Warm-hearted
Dry-spirited	Sweet-spirited
Erotic-presence	Strong-spirited
Free-spirited	Hard-hearted
Mean-spirited	Loving-spirited

PART THREE: YOUR SPIRIT'S HEALTH

6- HEALTH, SPIRITUAL HEALTH, AND SPIRITUAL HYGIENE

You know how important your physical and mental health are. You know the names of physical and mental diseases. No doubt you've been sick and injured more than once.

You know about over-the-counter medications for physical pain, cuts, sprains, rashes, and bruises. Perhaps you know about herbs that improve mental clarity and memory. You also know how important healthy relationships are.

But, when it comes to your spiritual health, what do you know? Chances are high that you know little, if anything at all. Can you name one spiritual disease?

Have you ever been spiritually ill or injured? Are there therapies for your spirit?

Your ignorance of spiritual health is not your fault. No one taught you. No one *could* teach you, not in Western culture anyway.

In Western culture, knowledge of spirit is ignored. It's associated with and overshadowed by faith in Spirit; that is, by faith in an invisible divine being and realm outside the scope of human science.

The point is not to deny faith in *capital 'S' Spirit*. The point is to reaffirm knowledge of *lower-case 's' spirit* and the importance of its health. The health of your spirit is every bit as important, if not more, as the health of your body, mind, and relationships.

Health

The word "healthy" means "whole." When you are healthy, you are whole. You are one. All your parts are integrated and working together in a harmonious whole.

You're healthy when your heart, hands, head, and homies all hum together in harmony. In other words, your spirit, body, mind, and relationships synchronize and function together as one. When all of your spiritual, physical, and mental parts are whole and functioning well in relationships with others, you are of sound spirit, body, mind, and relationships. You are healthy.

Spiritual Health

But what does it mean to be of sound spirit? What does it mean to be spiritually whole and healthy? You're spiritually healthy when all of the parts of your spirit are integrated, whole, working together, and fulfilling its purpose to make you alive and realize your joy.

Your spirit's *instincts* are driving you to do what you need to do to stay healthy and keep living. Its *emotions and moods* are alerting you to what is and isn't healthy for your spirit and life. Your spirit's *inner-tutor* is guiding you to do what is safe and avoid harm. Your spirit's *character* serves your life well in relationships with others. Your spirit contributes to the health of the larger spiritual wholes you are a smaller part of. Those larger wholes also contribute to your spirit's health.

When your body, mind, and relationships support the health of your spirit, and you are fulfilling its *life-affirming desires* and realizing your *joy*, you are healthy.

Spiritual Hygiene

"Hygiene" comes from the Ancient Greek phrase *hygiene techne*, meaning "the healthful technique or art." It could also be translated as "living well."

You know and practice basic physical hygiene: dress appropriately for the weather, wash your hands, brush your teeth, and cover your mouth when you cough. Cleanse and bandage cuts, and clean and put ointment on burns. Eat healthy food, stay hydrated, exercise, rest, and get enough sleep.

You know and practice basic psycho-social hygiene: Smile. Keep a positive attitude. Consider different points of view. Be willing to learn. Help those in need. Say, "Please" and "Thank you." Don't interrupt and so on.

What about hygiene for your spirit and the spirits of others? Have your learned spiritual hygiene? Has anyone taught you? Probably not.

The mindfulness of spirit exercise that you learned earlier is the essential practice of spiritual hygiene. It nurtures the health and wellness of your spirit. Just as you brush your teeth, strive to keep a positive attitude, and practice good manners daily, do the mindfulness of spirit exercise daily.

The five exercises presented in the next chapter expand your mindfulness to the spirits of others.

7- Five Spiritual Exercises

Spiritual Exercise #2: Connecting Spirit-to-Spirit with Others, Eyes Closed

The first spiritual exercise is mindfulness of your own spirit. Practicing it helps with the second spiritual exercise in which you become more aware of the spirits of others. As your spirit makes you alive, the spirits of others make them alive too.

As your instincts, emotions, moods, character traits, and heart-knowledge are of your spirit, so they are of the spirits of all living things. As you can physically touch or be of the same mind with others, so you can connect with others spirit-to-spirit.

Purpose

The purpose of this exercise is to be mentally aware

of your spirit-to-spirit connection with others. It's to turn your mind's attention to the spirits of others, with complete openness, full acceptance, and kind curiosity, and calmly hold your attention there with no expectations of outcomes.

Resources

As with the first fundamental exercise, you need nothing special to do this exercise. You already have everything you need.

Benefits

This exercise, like the first, uses your mind to serve your spirit. It heightens your mental awareness of your spirit-to-spirit connections with others. It affirms, heals, and strengthens your own spirit, the spirits of others, and your relationships with others. These benefits increase as you practice this exercise on a regular basis.

What to Do

1. Close your eyes and put your hands over your breastbone, the center of your chest.

2. Focus your mind's attention behind your breastbone. This is the heart of your being and center of your spirit. Smile at your own spirit.

3. When you breathe in, smile into your heart; when you breathe out, smile out of your heart.

4. When your mind wanders, simply return your attention to your heart. Breathe in and smile into your heart. Breathe out and smile out from your heart.

5. With your mind's attention still focused on your heart imagine, think about, and name the one you want to connect with spirit-to-spirit. With your mind hold them there in your heart.

6. Breathe in and smile to them in your heart; breathe out and smile to them in your heart.

7. If you become aware of things about the one you hold in your heart, form no opinions, just be together, connected, spirit-to-spirit.

8. Continue for as long as you like.

Spiritual Exercise #3: Connecting Spirit-to-Spirit, Eyes Open

After you feel comfortable connecting spirit-to-spirit with your eyes closed, practice connecting spirit-to-spirit with your eyes open. Entertain the idea that everything that moves is spirited and alive.

Physicists have been reporting for quite some time that everything is in constant motion. Everything is moving. Take that one step further: everything is spirited, alive.

Try connecting spirit-to-spirit with others besides humans. If you have pets, try connecting with them. Try connecting with plants in your home and outside. Tree hugging is optional. Find an interesting rock or gemstone and connect with it. Be open to whatever you experience. It's okay if you experience nothing unusual at all.

Experiment with connecting spirit-to-spirit with a stream, creek, river, waterfall, lake, or ocean. Try connecting with the wind you feel on your face and in your hair. Mountains, valleys, and other landforms are also fascinating to connect with. Try connecting with the sun, moon, planets, and stars.

What do you experience? How do they feel to you? How does it feel to connect spirit-to-spirit? What did you learn?

Add practicing this basic exercise to your day, develop your skill, and see where it takes you.

Exercise #4: How to Avoid Spiritual Harm: Inspired Action

Your three-basic mindfulness of spirit exercises are foundational: mindfulness of your own spirit, connecting spirit-to-spirit with others, with your eyes closed and open. The following practices of spiritual hygiene build on them. They support the health and well-being of your spirit.

The most important practice of spiritual hygiene is *inspired action.* It's the practice of *attending to and going with the guidance of your inner-tutor and guardian.* When you practice inspired action, you avoid harm, live a healthier life, and engage in realizing your joy. You waste less time due to "forgetting" something, taking a route that is congested or blocked, agreeing to do something that harms you, and other unwise actions.

Practicing inspired action requires trust. You must trust your inner-tutor. That trust builds as you practice inspired action instead of rationalizing away the guidance of your own spirit. Avoid what your inner-tutor prompts you to avoid. Go where it inspires you to go. Learn to discern the difference between your spirit's inner guidance and your mind's memories of what you've been taught, what you've experienced, and what seems logical.

Exercise #5: How to Nourish Your Spirit: Pause for Beauty

Perhaps you've seen bumper stickers that say, "I brake for dogs" or something similar. The practice introduced in this section is related. It's about pausing for beauty. There was a time when the pace of life allowed time for our natural response of *pausing for beauty*. That time is gone.

Today the hurried pace of life—with its stress, narrowed field of vision, and prolonged screen time—filters out most of the beauty around us. These days you must be intentional about being on alert and pausing for beauty. You must choose to slow down, stop, and take beauty in.

Why bother? Why pause for beauty? It nourishes, uplifts, heals and renews your spirit. Pausing for beauty is to your spiritual hygiene what staying hydrated is to your physical hygiene.

Pausing for beauty is slowing down or stopping to take in a moment of *visual* beauty: an attractive person, a remarkable dog, a bluebird, a fantastic photograph or painting, a dandelion blooming in the crack of a sidewalk, a stunning old oak tree, a cloud, a brilliant sunrise or sunset, or the bright silver moon.

It's slowing down or stopping for a moment of

beautiful *sound*: a sparrow's song, crickets chirping, children laughing, a talented street musician, the baritone growl of a Mustang's customized muffler, the sounds of neighbor's in the throes of sexual passion.

Moments of beauty might be the *aromas* of bread or cookies baking, patchouli essential oil, fresh blooming honeysuckle or roses, your lover's body, or some other arresting fragrance.

Touches are also moments of beauty: a silk tie, plush sweater, the soft fur of a cat or dog, a loved one's hair, a baby's cheek, a warm blanket from the dryer, your lover's bare skin cuddled against yours.

Moments of beauty also come in *tastes*: rich morning coffee or tea, fresh blueberries and strawberries, richly seasoned meatloaf, delicious wine, fine bourbon, creamy chocolate, your lover's lips and other parts.

Your *memory and ability to fantasize* are mental sources of beauty. Pause every now and then to recall moments of feeling joy. Take time to imagine your dreams coming true. Moments of beauty occur in *conversations and activities with others* as well. Be fully present. Absorb them. They increase your cache of memories to enjoy in the future.

Exercise #6: How to Cleanse Your Spirit

You're human. Your knowledge and abilities are limited. Expecting to never make mistakes and shaming yourself when you do, is more than unrealistic. It's cruel. Interacting with people who are harmful, or toxic is unavoidable. You don't always go with your inner-tutor. Your inner-tutor isn't right 100% of the time.

So, you must know how to cleanse your spirit. Cleansing your spirit is to your spirit what bathing is to your body. As bathing (hydrotherapy) helps you recover from physical trauma, cleansing your spirit enables you to recover from emotional distress. As bathing removes dirt and oil from your body, spiritual cleansing clears "ickiness" from your spirit that infects it after interacting with someone toxic.

Cleansing Your Spirit

After two or three minutes of practicing your essential mindfulness of spirit exercise…

1. Breathe in through your nose and lift your crossed hands away from your breastbone.

2. Blow your breath out through your mouth, and with your right hand, sweep the air in front of your heart downward and outward to your right.

3. Breathe in through your nose and raise your left hand up slightly above your heart.

4. Blow your breath out through your mouth, and with your left hand, sweep the air in front of your heart downward and outward to your left.

5. Repeat the sweeping motion with your right and left hands at least three times.

NOTE: When you blow your breath out and sweep with your hand, do so to clear and cleanse your heart and spirit.

Cleansing your spirit after you come home from interacting with others in public is an excellent practice. Stepping away to a private place and cleansing your spirit after a toxic interaction during your day is also excellent spiritual hygiene.

Nurture Your Spirit's Prosperity

In Western culture today, prosperity is often measured by how much an individual consumes. It is associated with financial resources, buying power, accumulating things, and consuming commodities and services. The more you collect and consume, the more prosperous you are.

It hasn't always been that way. Not long ago, prosperity was measured by how consistently you produced high-quality goods and services; the more consistently you produced those, the more prosperous you were.

Why? Because value was placed in consistent productivity and high quality rather than paying the lowest price. An abundant crop of high-quality strawberries was valued, prized, and gladly negotiated for. An abundance of unique, well-crafted, handsome furniture created a favorable reputation and attracted customers, who happily paid for what they received.

Prospering, consistently producing high-quality goods and services, is itself the fruit of a healthy and fertile spirit. All the spiritual practices presented in this book nurture the prosperity of your spirit. To quote a wise blessing familiar to Star Trek fans, "Live long and prosper!"

PART FOUR: SPIRITUAL DISEASE AND HEALING

8- DISEASE, SPIRITUAL DISEASE, SPIRITUAL HEALING

Health is not your default condition. In spite of your best hygienic efforts, your health varies. That it varies is normal and natural. You're human: you change, grow, develop, suffer illnesses and injuries, recover your health, and repeat the cycle. Eventually, you decline, die, and disintegrate.

You experience physical diseases: physical weaknesses, limitations, illnesses, and injuries. You experience mental diseases: confusion, memory loss, recurring disturbing memories, unwanted thoughts and imaginings, other conflicting thoughts, and troubling beliefs.

You know social dis-ease: failures to communicate, conflicts, abuse, neglect, violations of personal boundaries, alienations, and broken relationships. At times, you suffer from financial, food, clothing, shelter, and transportation insecurities.

What about your spirit? Are you aware of diseases of your spirit? Probably not, and it's not your fault. No one taught you. No one taught you because spiritual illness and injury are ignored in Western culture today. As mentioned earlier, it's associated with, and overshadowed by, belief in an invisible, divine Spirit. It's also conflated with mental disorders and obscured.

What is Spiritual Disease?

If your instincts have failed you, if you've lost your healthy appetite, sleep pattern, sexual desire, interest in caring for yourself, or desire to live, then you've suffered spiritual disease. If you've ever felt weak, weary with life, apathetic, heartache, or broken hearted, then you know spiritual disease first-hand. You've probably seen it in others too.

Chronic moods such as depression, anxiety, and even bliss that interfere with activities of daily living are spiritual diseases. A wounded spirit is spiritual disease. A broken spirit is often deadly.

Perhaps you know someone who died from a broken "heart."

Your spirit is what makes you alive rather than not. It also makes you more or less alive at different times. When it's ill or injured, its ability to make you alive diminishes. When you expire (spirit out), you die. Your spirit, mind, relationships, and body separate from each other.

Your spirit dissipates into the wind. Your psyche flies free; it stops living but still exists. Your relationships remain and are forever changed. Your body decomposes and returns to the earth.

Spiritual Healing

Trees are responsible for their own health and well-being. Being responsible isn't about being held morally accountable. It's not about judgment, shaming, and punishment. Responsibility is about power. It's the *ability to respond*. Trees are *able to respond* for their spirit's health and well-being.

They push their roots deep into the ground for food and water. They spread their limbs and leaves toward the sunlight for nourishment. They breathe. The bear fruit and offspring. They shed leaves that no longer serve them and rest for the winter.

Everything they do sustains their spirit and life. As they sustain their own spirit and life, they sustain the spirits and lives of others too. Everyone benefits.

You are responsible for your own spirit and life. You have the power, the *ability to respond* for your own spirit's health and well-being. It's up to you to invest some of your power into the health and well-being of your spirit. As you do, you not only sustain your own spirit and life, you sustain all others as well.

When you suffer with a spiritual illness or injury, you are *able to respond* for your healing. You have that power. You are your primary health care provider. You are the first responder to your illness or injury. You see your recovery through to its completion.

When your recovery is beyond your ability to complete by yourself, and you access professional help, you remain your primary health care provider. All others work for you. They give second opinions that help you decide what to do to support your healing and recovery.

Healing

Healing is the process of reintegrating, becoming integrated and whole again.

Physically, it's the process of a broken bone mending and becoming whole again, a cut finger flushing with blood, scabbing, and mending. It's the process of neutralizing or removing harmful bacteria, viruses, and toxic tissue that is too damaged to heal.

Mentally, healing is the process of reintegrating the mind and its functions of processing language, remembering, imagining, problem-solving, and orientation to self, time, and place.

Socially, healing is about mending or ending broken relationships. It's also about securing basic needs for life: safety, food, clothing, shelter, transportation, and healthy relationships.

Spiritual healing is the process of reintegrating the spirit's instincts, emotions, moods, knowing, and character. It's about reawakening and nurturing instincts that support health and life, recovering from emotional wounds and broken hearts, and restoring trust in your spirit's inner-knowing and guidance.

Spiritual healing is essential to physical, mental,

and social healing because your spirit is the life of your body, mind, and relationships. Only with spirit are you physical, mentally, and socially alive. Without spirit, you're dead.

9- Natural Healing and How to Heal Your Spirit

Natural Response

Healing is a natural response. As soon as you're sick or injured physically, mentally, or socially, your natural healing response begins. The same is true of your spirit. As soon as your spirit is wounded or broken, it begins healing.

Healing isn't immediate; it takes time. In the pace of life today, it often takes longer than we like. Impatience with your healing is resistance to your natural healing response. It delays and prolongs your healing.

Acceptance of your need to take time to heal and patience with the process facilitates your healing. With acceptance and patience, you heal sooner. It's not true that time heals. Time itself does not heal, but healing takes time. It takes time for your body, mind, spirit, and relationships to reintegrate and become whole again.

Besides time, healing requires work. In other words, it requires therapy. Therapy and healing are two different processes. Healing is an automatic, natural process. Therapy is a choice that facilitates your natural healing process.

Therapy is attending to, serving, and taking care of your healing process. Just as you are your primary health care provider, you are your primary therapist. You are the first to attend to, serve, and care for your injury or illness. You also attend to, serve, and care for your healing process to its completion.

For example, therapy to help your body heal might require cleansing the wound and applying an ointment and a bandage. Therapy to help heal your mental confusion might require learning a different way of thinking about things.

Therapy for healing relationships might require learning how to improve your listening and communication skills. And, therapy for healing your spirit might require processing your emotions and moods by fully feeling them, identifying them, talking about them, resolving them, and taking constructive steps to get to a better place in life.

Exercise #7: How to Heal Your Spirit

You know basic first aid and therapy practices that facilitate physical, mental, and relational healing. Here is a basic practice for healing your spirit. It's called Heart-Centered Self-Healing.

Setting

- Solitude

- Quiet

- Safe from interruptions for 30 minutes

- Comfortable posture

Preparation

Do your mindfulness of spirit practice for two or three minutes:

1. Cross hands over your breastbone.

2. Focus attention beneath your hands and behind your breastbone, in your heart.

3. Breathe in/breathe out: "I smile into my heart/I smile out from my heart."

4. Keep your hands crossed over your heart and your attention focused in it.

5. Continue breathing a smile into and out from your heart.

6. Repeat each step below three or more times.

Practice

1. *Acknowledge:* Breathe in. Breathe out and say aloud or in your heart, "I have a problem."

2. *Name:* Breathe in. Breathe out and say, "I have a problem with ______."

3. *Thank your spirit:* Breathe in. Breathe out and say, "Thank you for bringing this problem to my awareness."

4. *Locate the problem:* Breathe in. Breathe out and say, "This problem is in me."

5. *Own your problem:* Breathe in. Breathe out and say, "I take 100% responsibility for my problem with ______."

6. *Suspend analyzing:* Breathe in. Breathe out and say, "I suspend analyzing why I have this problem."

7. *Breathe:* Breathe in and say, "I breathe into my problem. Breathe out and say, "I breathe out of my problem."

8. *Feel and name your emotion(s):* fear, sadness, anger, guilt, disappointment, disgust, etc.

   Breathe in. Breathe out and say, "I feel the _____ in my problem with _____."

9. *Release:* Breathe in. Breathe out and say, "I release my (emotion); I let it fly free."

10. *Affirm your spirit's life-affirming desire:* Breathe in. Breathe out and say, "Now I am free to _______!"

When You Need Professional Help

Sometimes your healing requires more knowledge and skill than you, your family, and friends have. That's okay. You're human. So are your family and friends. You all have limits.

Sometimes your automotive and plumbing needs require more knowledge and skill than you and your family and friends have too. As with other needs, when your healing requires more knowledge and skill than you have available, you contact the appropriate professional for help.

For physical healing, you see your physician and/or physical therapist. For mental healing, you see a psychotherapist. For social support, you see social workers.

Unfortunately, no network of professionals who provide therapy for spiritual healing yet exists; not as it is described here. I am the only provider as of the publication of this book.

Please see my contact information in the back of this book for a free discovery consultation. I see clients in person and online through a secure platform.

Remember, any professional therapist you partner with joins with you in attending to, serving, and caring for you in your healing process. You are your primary health care provider. Your therapist works for you.

PART FIVE: HOW TO KNOW YOUR REASON FOR BEING ALIVE

10-QUESTIONS AND A QUEST

Your spirit's health serves a purpose beyond itself. It serves your reason for being alive.

You're not alive just to live. You're alive for a reason. You're alive to accomplish something only you can. You're alive to realize your dream. Your dream is your joy. Nothing, absolutely nothing is more critical for you to do than realize your joy.

To realize your joy, you must know what it is. Nothing is more critical for you to know. When you know your joy, your life has a direction. You live toward your joy. Your joy is your North Star, GPS, lighthouse, and landmark.

Every action you take is related to your joy. Every step either contributes to realizing your joy or detracts from it. So, how do you know your joy? That's a question you yourself answer. No one else tells you what your joy is or how to know it. However, some clues might help.

Your joy is what you're here to do. It's your dream to realize. Your joy might be to bring something new into the world: a solution to a problem, a discovery, a work of art, or something else.

Or, your joy might be to work on realizing something others worked on before you were born and will work on after you die. It will be realized in the future, and you play an essential role in the process: the search for life elsewhere in the universe, a cure for Alzheimer's disease, a grand work of architecture, understanding animal communication, the end of government corruption, or something else. In other words, your joy could be either a point of completion or engaging in a process.

How do you know? Here are some questions to consider:

1. *If you had health and unlimited wealth, what would you do with your time and energy?*

2. *What have you imagined doing for as long as you can remember?*

3. *What comes naturally to you that others either cannot do or struggle to do?*

4. *What problem do you see that attracts you emotionally and you desire to solve?*

5. *What do you do, that when you do it, you lose track of time?*

6. *What kind of work do you do, that when you do it, you feel energized?*

7. *What are the life-affirming desires of your heart?*

In addition to self-reflection, talk with several others who have known you for a while. Ask them what they see in you.

Try a Vision Quest

A vision quest might help you become mentally aware of your dream and joy. A vision quest is

nothing exotic unless you want it to be. It's a get-
away.

Leave your everyday surroundings and routine. Go
somewhere different with the sole intention of
becoming aware of your dream.

Go where you can focus and won't be distracted or
interrupted. Give yourself two or three days.

Take a journal and pen. Handwriting is better for
this than a computer. Take the questions listed
above.

Set your intention to know your joy. Practice the
essential mindfulness of spirit exercise.

Read each question and allow time for your answers
to arise from within. Suspend your expectations of
what will happen.

Attend to the sights and sounds around you as well.
Something might feel like a sign. Take it in.

Be open and receptive to whatever emerges from
within and catches your attention in your
surroundings.

Attend more to your heart, emotions, and inner
knowing than to your mental self-talk. Watch for
images that appear spontaneously in your mind's
eye.

Trust that when you become aware of your dream, your spirit will alert you to with an emotional "Yes!"

After becoming aware of your dream, make a vision boa rd. Imagine how your joy realized looks in the world. Make a visual representation of it.

Make your visual representation of your joy realized in the world as simple or elaborate as you want. It serves you and no one else. It's for your eyes only. Look at it often and let it guide your actions to realize it.

CONCLUSION

Knowing your spirit is one thing. Living from your spirit is another. Now that you know more about your own spirit and the spirits of others, it's time to practice what you know.

Practice the mindfulness of spirit exercises alone frequently. Then practice being mindful of your own and other's spirits as you are with them and make your way through each day. Practice trusting and acting in accord with your instincts. Practice being aware of your emotions and identifying them. Consciously determine which emotions are mind-based and which are experience-based.

Observe your moods. When do they begin? How long do they last? When do they end?

Practice inspired action, attending to and going with your inner-tutor's guidance.

How would you describe the character of your spirit?

How would you describe the character of the spirits of others you know?

Practice good spiritual hygiene.

Most importantly, fulfill the life-affirming desires of your heart and realize your joy.

You must fulfill the life-affirming desires of your heart and realize your joy.

Do it for yourself and everyone else too.

Looking Ahead

If you're hungry for more spiritual knowledge, read my first book *Re-Visioning Spirit: A Brief Introduction to Thumotics*. There you will learn more about your spirit, spiritual knowledge, loving care of spirit, spiritual healing, spirituality, and spiritual community.

For developing life-affirming self-talk, see my book *Affirmations of Life.*

Also, watch for two books that lay the theoretical and practical foundations for a new science and therapy of spirit: *Your Life: An Owner's Manual* and *Life Therapy: A Phenomenal View of Life.*

THE THUMOTIC MANIFESTO

Vision

I believe in a world where more of us are healthy and whole, fulfilling the life-affirming desires of our hearts, and realizing our dreams.

When I say "I believe" in such a world, I don't mean I have blind faith in it. I mean that I am actively putting my trust in and relying on such a world. It means I'm personally engaged in making such a world real.

When I say I believe in a world where "more of us are healthy and whole", I mean all living things, not just humans. I don't mean disease-free. I don't mean without suffering. I mean that we have integrity; that our hearts, hands, heads, and homies all hum together in harmony.

When I say I believe in a world where more of us are "fulfilling the life-affirming desires of our hearts," I mean that we know why we're here. We know our reason for being alive. We are doing what we're here to do and not letting anything stop us. What we're doing is good for us and everybody else too.

When I say I believe in a world where more of us are "realizing our dreams," by dreams I mean joy. When we are fulfilling the life-affirming desires of our hearts and making them visible in this world, we shine bright with joy. Others light up with joy too.

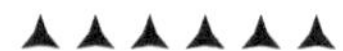

SPIRIT

Essential to realizing this vision of the world is *spirit*. Our spirit is necessary for our life, health and wholeness. Only by our spirit are we alive. Our spirit is what makes and keeps us alive. The health of our spirit is the health of our body, mind, and relationships.

Heart is another word for spirit. The life-affirming desires of our hearts are the life-affirming desires of our own *spirits*.

The dreams we're here to realize are the joys of our own spirits.

Thumos

I call this manifesto "Thumotic" because it is about re-visioning spirit in the light of the Ancient Greek word *thumos*.

Thumos was well-known by Greeks for about two thousand years, from around 1200 BCE to around 600

CE. Homer used *thumos* over seven hundred times in his epic songs, the *Iliad* and the *Odyssey*. Hesiod, Sappho, and other poets sang of *thumos* too. *Thumos* played essential roles in the tragedies and comedies of Aeschylus and the other dramatic poets.

Even the Greek historians and Hippocrates, the father of Western medicine, spoke of *thumos* like the poets did before them. All who heard the poets' rhymed and metered songs knew what *thumos* referred to. It referred to a natural phenomenon, the natural force that made all living things alive. Not only humans, but the goddesses and gods, and many things that we now believe to be inanimate had *thumos*.

The Roman poets, especially Virgil, assimilated *thumos* into Latin as *spiritus*, from which we now have *spirit*. Western culture, deeply rooted in Ancient Greek and Roman culture, is profoundly influenced by Ancient Greek words like psyche, logos, soma, bios, and polis, but not *thumos*. Why?

Spirit in Western Culture

Influenced by Middle Eastern religious ideas, Socrates, Plato, and Aristotle corrupted the indigenous Greek understanding of *thumos*. They devalued *thumos* and glorified psyche, logic, hyper-rationality, and other-worldly aspirations.

Roman philosophers assimilated Greek philosophy and kept its Middle Eastern religious ideas alive. Later, adherents of the Middle Eastern religion, Christianity, used Greco-Roman philosophy, especially the ideas of Socrates and Plato, to form Christian theology.

With the rise to dominance of Christianity, Westerners turned their attention away from experiencing the natural force of spirit to believing in the Christian Holy Spirit instead. They valued being filled and possessed by the supernatural Holy Spirit of their God. They ignored and devalued the natural force of spirit that makes living things alive.

While belief in the Holy Spirit dominated Western culture, knowledge of the natural force of spirit declined. The consequential ignorance of spirit, and the devaluing of life that went with it, devastated the lives and culture of Westerners.

Since the Renaissance occurred within the context of Christian dominance, Westerners missed the opportunity to include the natural force of spirit in the re-birth of Greco-Roman culture. The Protestant Reformation, and Roman Catholic Counter-Reformation reinforced the dominance of belief in the Holy Spirit and ongoing ignorance of the natural force of spirit.

In Modern Western and now Postmodern Western culture, belief in a divine Spirit remains popular. It has, however, become more diverse and diluted due to Eastern religious influences.

At the same time, growing numbers of Westerners identify as non-religious, agnostic, and atheist. Along with their rejection of belief in a divine Spirit, they also ignore the natural force of spirit.

Ignorance of the natural force of spirit remains the norm. It is at the heart of many problems in Western culture and throughout the world today.

Consequences of Ignoring Spirit

Ignorance of the natural force of spirit is ignorance of life. Ignorance of life is disregard of life itself. Evidence of Western disregard of life is as abundant as the formerly visible stars of the night sky. The evidence includes far more than the light and air pollution that now obscures our view of the stars dancing in the night sky.

It includes oppression, war, and other life-denying and deadly acts of violence against humans and all forms of life on Earth. It's evidenced by our life-denying pollution of the soil, air, and water on which our own lives and the lives of all living things depend. It's evidenced by our extinction of masses of our own kind and entire species of plants and animals.

This *Thumotic Manifesto* is about attending to and knowing again the natural force of spirit rather than continuing to ignore and remain ignorant of it. It is about completing the Renaissance by re-visioning spirit in the light of *thumos* as it was known in pre-Christian Greco-Roman culture. Knowing spirit again, as the natural force that makes living things alive, empowers us to re-vision spirit for today. Re-visioning spirit makes it possible for us to realize a new dream of our world. It's a dream of life, health, and fulfillment. It's a joy that we realize together.

Spirit Re-Visioned for Today

When we re-vision spirit in the light of *thumos,* we see
that our spirit is what makes us alive. And what a
profound mystery life is! What a profound mystery it is
that we are alive rather than not! And we are not alone.
We are alive together, with all other living things of this
world.

The spirit that makes us alive is our own. As we have
our own body and mind, we also have our own spirit. As
our body and mind have their own unique identities, so
does our spirit. Reducing our spirit to generic energy or
a chemical process, conflating it with our psyche or a
divine being, devalues, denies, and disregards the
independent status of our spirit's existence.

Our spirit exists with its own unique identity,
distinguishable from our body and mind. It is unique and
exists in its own right in each one of us. Our spirit is a
natural phenomenon, a force of nature similar to
magnetism, electricity, and other basic natural forces. As
these natural forces are energies organized in specific
ways that produce specific effects, spirit is energy
organized in a specific way that produces life.

As bodies and minds have their own anatomies and
functions, so do spirits. In us humans, the anatomy and
functions of our spirit include its *agency.* It not only
makes us alive; it compels us to keep living and remain
alive.

Our spirit's *instincts* compel us to do what we need to do

to stay alive. Our spirit's *emotional responses* alert us to
what affirms and denies our life. Our *moods* are our
spirit's extended emotions. Our heart-knowledge and
inner-knowing is our spirit's wordless cognizance. Our
spirit prompts many of our vocalizations. Our
personality and *character* are informed by our spirit.

The *life-affirming desires* of our spirits compel us to
realize our *dreams*. Every individual is spirited and alive
for a reason—to realize their dream and joy. Realizing
our dreams is essential to our health and well-being.

When we engage in fulfilling the life-affirming desires
of our hearts and realizing our dreams, we live healthier,
happier lives—lives that go well and inspire joy in our
own spirits and the spirits of others.

The natural force of spirit makes groups as well as
individuals alive. Families, teams, schools, businesses,
military units, nonprofit organizations, and countless
other social groups have their own spirits, their *esprit de
corps*.

Just as individual spirits have life-affirming desires to
fulfill and dreams to realize, so do the spirits of groups.
Just as individual spirits have their own anatomies and
personalities, so do the spirits of groups.

MISSION

This manifesto is about inciting and organizing a
movement of spirit-centered individuals and groups who

have as their mission *creating a world where more of us
are healthy and whole, fulfilling the life-affirming
desires of our hearts, and realizing our dreams.*

Those who participate in this movement re-vision spirit
for today in the light of *thumos*. They share a consensus
that spirit refers to the natural phenomenon and force
that makes living things alive. In their own ways, they
engage in realizing the vision of this *Thumotic
Manifesto*.

VALUES

To realize their mission, the individuals and groups in
this movement practice and embody these seven values:

1. *Spirit*

We value spirit as re-visioned for today in the light of
thumos. We share a consensus that the word spirit refers
to the natural force that makes living things alive. We
recognize that both individuals and groups have their
own spirits. *Esprit de corps* is a natural phenomenon we
acknowledge. This manifesto describes the *esprit de
corps* of the movement it instigates. We propose that
Westerners and others adopt the clear definition of spirit
we share in this manifesto.

We believe that sharing a consensus on the meaning of
spirit makes possible:

- A broader cultural consensus on what the word spirit refers to
- Coherent public conversations about spirit
- Sciences devoted to studying the natural force of spirit
- Historical study of spirit in Western and other cultures
- A growing, publicly shared body of knowledge about spirit
- Knowledge of the health of spirit
- Knowledge of the diseases of spirit
- Hygienic practices for nurturing healthy spirits
- Primary education for children about spirit
- Therapies for caring for diseased spirits
- University and college degrees and other academic programs devoted to spirit
- Credentialed and licensed professionals devoted to the care of spirit
- Laws protecting the safety of spirit

2. *Life*

We value the life that spirit is and makes possible.

We value not only human life, but all life.

We understand life to be an animating force, condition, time-period, and narrative.

Life is an *animating force*. All living things have life in them. Life is another word for spirit.

Life is the *condition* of being alive rather than not. It is the condition of being spirited. All living things have in common the condition of being spirited and alive.

Life is a *time-period*. For humans, life is the time period from birth to death. It is marked by our birth and death dates. We are never more human and alive than during our lifetime. Whether human life begins before birth and continues after death remains open to discussion.

Life is a *narrative*. It is the story represented by the dash between our birth and death dates. For us humans, it is the story of our lifetime told as either autobiography or biography. Informally, it is our reputation, the stories others tell about us. Our name is an abbreviation for our life-story. With our life-story we make a name for ourselves.

3. *Wonder*

We value wonder. We open our hearts and minds to both *being wondered by* the mere fact of being alive and *wondering about* the mystery of being alive. We are wondered by and wonder about the mere fact of, not only human life, but the lives of all living things.

4. *Freedom*

We value freedom. Freedom is self-determination. It's living our life as we choose. It includes the opportunity to set one's own boundaries and limits.

Freedom is not absolute. It is limited by valuing and respecting the spirits and lives of others. It allows others the same self-determination.

Exceptions to violating another's freedom include self-defense and sustaining one's own life as well as the lives of others in one's care.

5. *Tolerance*

We value tolerance. Far from laxity or passivity, tolerance is strength. It is the ability to allow for diversity and differences. Tolerance secures freedom.

It respects the freedom of others to determine their own lives. It accepts the freedom of others without agreeing with their choices.

Tolerance is the opposite of xenophobia, the fear and rejection of those unfamiliar to us.

6. *Health and Healing*

We value health. Health is wholeness. It is not our default condition. It varies. Disease is as much an experience of life as is health.

We value healing. Healing is a natural process. It often happens with little or no effort at all. However, sometimes our natural healing process requires assistance.

We value all therapists who assist with healing and restoring our ability to live, fulfill our heart's desires, and realize our dreams.

Since spirit is what makes us alive, its health precedes and determines the health of our body, mind, relationships, and social groups.

The health and healing of individual and collective spirits have long been ignored and neglected in Western culture. Because of this fact, we especially value efforts to understand the health, disease, and healing of spirits as well as therapies for ill and injured spirits.

7. *Realization of Dreams*

We value the realization of individual and group dreams. Realizing our individual and group dreams *as humans* is our reason for being alive. It is the reason for *every* living thing to be alive.

Every individual and group has a dream, a joy, to realize. The life-affirming desires of our hearts compel us to realize our dreams and joys. Our dreams themselves draw us to realize them.

▲▲▲▲▲▲▲

ORGANIZATION OF THE MOVEMENT

Instigator

The instigator of the movement described in this manifesto is Mark W. Neville. The vision, mission, and values presented here as well as the call to join the movement were first articulated by him.

First Associates

The first associates are those who first join the movement and help to establish and organize it into an identifiable movement. All who join the movement after the publication of the first by-laws are associates.

Leading Associates

Leading Associates are those who lead subgroups in realizing their designated aspects of the grand vision described in this manifesto.

Associates

All who join in this movement to realize the vision described in the manifesto are Associates.

Friends

Friends of this movement are all who share in whole or in part the mission, vision, and values of this movement. We gladly seek and welcome opportunities to partner with individuals, movements, and organizations to facilitate the realization of shared interests.

Foes

The foes of this movement are those who oppose the vision, mission, and values of this movement. We welcome and tolerate opposition and express our deep gratitude for our foes. Without them, this movement would have no reason to exist. Our foes make us necessary.

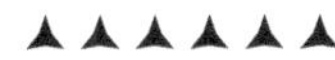

CALL TO JOIN

This manifesto is your invitation to join with others in an organized movement to re-vision spirit in the light of *thumos* and reclaim it for today. It is your invitation to acknowledge, affirm, heal, sustain, and fulfill your own life-giving spirit as well as the life-giving spirits of all other living things.

This is your invitation to engage in realizing a vision of this world where more of us are fulfilling the life-affirming desires of our hearts and realizing our unique, individual and group dreams.

To accept this invitation contact me at www.markwneville.com

 Join with everyone else engaged in this movement to create a world where more of us are healthy and whole, fulfilling our hearts' life-affirming desires, and realizing our dreams and joys.

From my heart to yours,

Mark W. Neville

Mark W. Neville
Instigator

ABOUT THE AUTHOR

Mark W. Neville is the originator of Life Therapy as well as a thought-leader, author, and educator. He lives with Lisa—his best friend, lover, and wife—in Hendersonville, NC where they enjoy their life together in the natural beauty of the Southern Appalachian Mountains. Trees have a special place in their hearts.

Mark formed Life Therapy, a holistic alternative to modern medication therapy and psychotherapy, out of his formal education, personal life experiences, and over thirty years of counseling individuals, couples, and families through life's most difficult challenges. For over ten years he worked for a nationally awarded, nonprofit hospice organization where he served as the Director of Counseling Services and counselor.

He now has a private practice and cares for clients in his offices in Asheville and Hendersonville as well as online via a secure platform.

Mark is the author of three blogs—*Mindful of Spirit, Life Therapy with Mark*, and *Your Spirit, Your Life*—and the books in the *Your Spirit, Your Life* series: *Re-Visioning Spirit: A Brief Introduction to Thumotics* and *Affirmations of Life* (includes *The Thumotic Manifesto)*.

For more information, to schedule an appointment, join the movement to re-vision spirit, or purchase his books visit www.markwneville.com

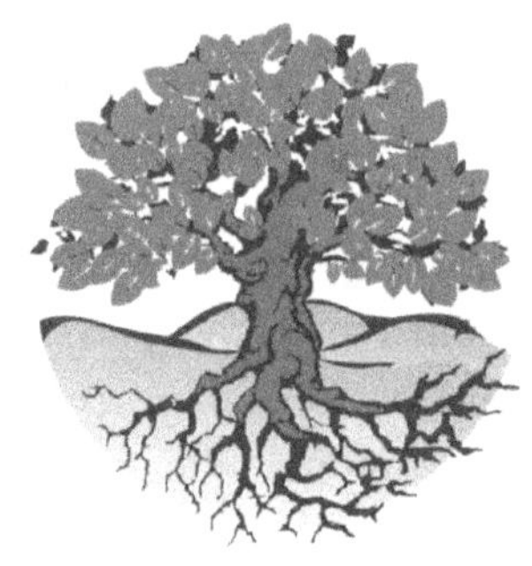

www.ingramcontent.com/pod-product-compliance
Lightning Source LLC
Chambersburg PA
CBHW071019260726
48662CB00022B/612